LOSING WEIGHT THE EASY WAY:

Learning Healthy Ways To Weight Lose

Bennie Haskins

TABLE OF CONTENT

Chapter 1

WEIGHT AND HEALTH

Being overweight or obese raises our risk of several ailments. The research in a certain nation suggests that roughly 75% of men and 60% of women are carrying too much body fat and 25% of youngsters are overweight or obese. This implies the incidence of obesity-related illnesses (such as coronary heart disease and diabetes), is also on the increase. Losing weight has become a multi-billion-dollar business. It's impossible to spend a day without seeing or hearing about 'the answer to' or a 'miracle' weight-loss treatment.

The practical way to decrease extra body fat is to make minor healthy modifications to your food and activity routines. These modifications should be something that you can sustain as part of your lifestyle, that way you will lose weight and keep it off.

However, there are numerous misunderstandings regarding reducing weight. Popular media is full of fad diets and miracle weight reduction potions advocated by celebrities and backed by personal success stories. While many of these diets may assist you to lose weight while you're following them, as soon as you resume your ordinary lifestyle, the weight begins to creep back on. That's because losing weight isn't necessarily the difficulty, it's keeping it off longer term that is challenging.

Managing your weight is a life-long commitment , not simply following a diet for a few weeks to reduce kg. Remember, if the methods you're putting into place to lose weight are not techniques that you'll be able to follow for the rest of your life, odds are you'll regain whatever weight you lose.

Most individuals believe dieting is the greatest method to weight reduction, without recognizing the damage it may bring them in the long term.

Dieting may be hazardous because our body reacts to these periods of semi-starvation by reducing its metabolic rate. When you lose weight too rapidly, you lose fat and muscle. Muscle burns kilojoules, while fat doesn't. So, after you quit dieting and return to your typical routines, your body will burn even fewer calories than before since the relative amount of muscle in your body has dropped and your metabolic rate is slower.

This sort of eating behavior may also damage our overall health,in that just one cycle of weight loss and weight gain can lead to an elevated risk of coronary heart disease (independent of our body fat levels) (regardless of our body fat levels). That's why it's more crucial to be able to sustain weight reduction. Weight reduction of roughly half (½) to 1kg per week is regarded as normal and more likely to be sustained.

There are many harmful beliefs about weight reduction but to lower your weight, and keep it off, you need to make tiny, doable adjustments to your lifestyle. If you are carrying extra weight, modifying the way you eat and increasing your physical activity, in a manner that you can stay with over the longer term, is the greatest approach to lose and maintain weight reduction.

To keep a steady weight, your energy (kilojoule) intake has to match the energy you utilize. If you burn more energy than you ingest, you will lose weight. On the other hand, if you consume more than you utilize, you will gain weight.

Small imbalances over lengthy periods of time might lead you to become overweight or obese. The main thing is to have a balanced diet and eat enough nutrient packed meals. It is also vital to restrict the number of calorie packed, nutrition poor meals to have a healthy weight.

Chapter 2

STARTING THE WEIGHT LOSS PLAN

One thing to know about weight reduction is that it is not miraculous, rather it is a consequence of work channeled in the appropriate road towards maintaining a healthy and balanced weight. It's easy to feel overwhelmed by all the information accessible. If you want to reduce weight, a smart start would be to base your diet on the guide to healthy eating. Avoiding unexpected or habitual eating, and adhering to regular meals and snacks, can also assist you to lose weight. It is also advised that if you have been on crash diets for many years or finding it tough, you may seek guidance from a dietician.

Dietitians can lead you to a healthy way of eating that is based on the latest research and adapted to fit your health and lifestyle. If you are overweight, over 40 years of age, or haven't exercised consistently for a long time, check with your doctor before you start any physical activity.

Understand your existing eating and exercise habits.Through the process of keeping a healthy weight, being careful of what we take as input and how we put it to use in exercise.

Once you have chosen to lose weight, it's a good idea to grasp your existing situation, that is what are your food and activity habits?

A smart approach to accomplish this is to break them into 'energy in' (diet) and 'energy out' (movement) (movement).

What energy (diet) are you taking in?

Take some time to think about your eating behaviors. Think about:

•What you consume.
•When you eat.
•Why do you eat.
•Keep a food journal

You may find it beneficial to maintain a food journal for a week to see if you can spot any trends or themes in your eating habits. Food diaries are best written at the moment (rather than at the end of the day) because there's less likely that you'll forget something:

•Write down everything you eat and drink.
•How you are feeling?
•Your hunger level at the moment.
Be as honest as possible. Try not to modify your behaviors, adjusting things is the next stage.
Your journal can begin to indicate a trend, such as you pick specific meals or beverages based on where you are or how you are feeling.

Recognize behaviors that contribute to weight gain
Some of the food-related practices that might contribute to weight gain include:

• Night eating — nibbling throughout the evening.
• Social eating — eating while in a gathering of friends or relatives.
• Emotional eating — eating in reaction to your emotions, whether it be boredom, exhaustion, worry, tension, joy, or despair.

• Distracted eating — eating whilst doing anything else (such as watching TV, working at your computer, or being on social media) (such as watching TV, working at your desk, or being on social media).

Read a book, phone a friend, or go for a stroll instead of nibbling when you are feeling depressed.
If you eat in front of the TV or at your computer, sit at a table and concentrate on the food you're eating, what are the colors, scents, tastes, and textures?
, by eating thoughtfully, you are more likely to appreciate food and will experience the impulse to quit eating when you're full.

The other side of the energy equation is the kilojoules you expend during movement. Not only does staying active burn energy, but it also inhibits muscle loss, which helps to maintain your metabolic rate ticking over at a healthy level. Just like maintaining a record of your food habits, you could also keep a diary for a week to monitor how much physical activity you're doing. Include episodes of physical exercise that last 10 minutes or longer. Break them into:

I Organised activities – such as walking, jogging, swimming, playing a sport, and cycling.

ii Incidental activities - such as gardening, housekeeping, standing at work, or moving heavy goods.

This can allow you to obtain an awareness of your current physical activity level and help you identify strategies to exercise more.
Once you understand your present patterns, the following stage is to determine how you will reduce weight.

Try to make your objectives SMART – be:
• Specific: write out precisely what you are aiming to accomplish. (For example, rather than I want to do more exercise, make it explicit that I will ride my bike to work on Monday and Wednesday.)
• Measurable – utilize numbers or quantities whenever feasible. (For example, I will consume 2 pieces of fruit, each day.)

• Achievable: there is no sense in setting down a goal that you will never accomplish. (For example, if you know you are unlikely to quit drinking on weekends, a better aim may be instead of having a glass of wine each weekday while watching my favorite tv show, I will drink a glass of water.)

• Realistic: your objective must to feasible and relevant to you. (For example, when I feel pressured, instead of munching, I will pause and ask myself why I feel this way. I will concentrate on this notion for 10 minutes to ascertain if I am hungry before I eat anything.)

• Time-bound: establish a time range for your objective to measure your progress. (For example, I will walk to work twice a week by the end of May.)

Remember, the best method to lose weight is to do it slowly by making tiny, manageable modifications to your diet and physical activity habits. You may wish to assign yourself one or 2 little adjustments to work on at a time, only adding to these once they have become your new way of life. Be nice to yourself, if things don't go according to plan, keep trying. You may need to change your objectives or the time it will take to attain them.

Staying motivated on the weight loss plan
Once you have a strategy in place, be realistic and attempt to concentrate on little wins to keep you on target. Some recommendations involve that you:

i. Don't depend on the numbers on the scales. Instead, measure your waist circumference, a healthy waist circumference is less than 94 cm for males and fewer than 80 cm for women.

ii. Notice how your clothes fit, maybe they feel loose, or you now fit into something that was hidden in the back of your closet.

iii. Become confident in an activity you've been avoiding (such as being able to keep up with the kids without becoming out of breath) (such as being able to keep up with the kids without getting out of breath).

Maybe you have more energy, things require less effort, or you are sleeping better. Losing and maintaining weight is a life-long commitment to a healthy lifestyle. Don't alter everything at once, a few tiny modifications to your food and activity, in the beginning, might make a major effect.

Make simple modifications to your diet (energy in), by decreasing body fat by adopting these few small changes to your eating habits:

i. Avoid crash and fad diets to reduce your risk of yoyo dieting.

ii. Try to consume a broad range of foods from all 5 food categories from the Australian Guide to Healthy Eating).

iii. Increase your fruit and vegetable consumption - especially veggies, which are low in kilojoules and include fiber, which helps you feel full.

iv. Be conscious of the amounts of meals and liquids you're eating - the greater the dish, the more energy it contains.

v. Reduce your consumption of foods that are heavy in added fat, saturated fat, sugar, and salt.

vi. Make soft beverages, sweets, snack items, and alcoholic drinks an occasional 'extra'.

vii. Most individuals should consume no more than one or 2 'treats' a day. If you are overweight or sedentary, you may need to restrict treats to fewer than one a day.
viii. Have a routine of eating and keep to it.
ix. Replace sugary beverages with water.

Try to balance an 'extra' meal with more activity. The more energy you expend, the more sweets you can afford to consume. Remember, you should only add additional foods once you have addressed your nutritional requirements with selections from the healthier food categories.
Don't remove any food group. Instead, pick from a broad variety of meals every day and prefer 'whole', less-processed foods. Also, avoid utilizing food for consolation, such as when you are unhappy, irritated, or anxious.

Explore alternative healthy strategies to deal with these sensations, (such as going for a walk, reading a book, taking a bath, or listening to music) (such as going for a walk, reading a book, having a bath, or listening to music).
Look at the facts, for instance, while it would be simple to eat a family-sized slab of chocolate in

one sitting, it will take 2.5 hours of running (or nearly 6 hours of walking) to burn off the energy it contains.

Simple methods to be more active (energy out) (energy out)

Although we may make excuses such as being too busy or fatigued, remember, that physical exercise does not have to be extremely demanding. Even modest quantities of physical exercise of approximately 30 minutes a day may speed up our metabolic rate and help us lose weight. We may also find ourselves less exhausted and have more energy to perform the activities we like.

When beginning off, take things gently. You may raise your activity levels by simply increasing movement throughout the day. The human body is meant for mobility and any physical exercise delivers advantages.

Try these basic suggestions:

• Incorporate moderate-intensity exercises throughout your day, such as going for a stroll, doing some gardening, or mowing the grass.

• If you drive to work, walk or ride your bike.

• If you need to drive, try to add some movement to your day. Park farther away or use public transit.

• While at work, talk to your coworkers in person rather than emailing them.

• If you spend most of the day sitting at work, get a stand-up desk or hold stand-up meetings.

• Go for a stroll at noon.

• When shopping, park farther away.

• Play a sport or perform an activity you like.

• Walk instead of using the vehicle on short journeys.

• Get off the train, bus, or tram one stop early and walk the rest of the way.

• Play more outdoor games with your family and friends.

• Walk the dog.

• Take stairs instead than elevators.

• Choose pleasurable hobbies, rather than ones you believe are beneficial for you. This provides you a higher chance of staying with them.

• Be imaginative - pick up an activity you loved as a youngster.

Keep things easy, you don't have to run a marathon (unless you want to) (unless you want to). Look for simple ways to be more active so you may start to boost the quantity of energy you burn, which will help you lose weight.

Chapter 3

THE FOOD NUTRIENT FOR ALL

Our nutritional demands fluctuate with various life stages. To stay fit and healthy, it is vital to take into consideration the increased demands put on your body by these changes.

To satisfy your body's normal nutritional demands, you should consume:

• A broad array of healthful foods.
• Water daily.
• Enough kilojoules for energy, with carbs being the preferable source.
• Essential fatty acids from meals such as oily fish, almonds, and avocado.
• Adequate protein for cell upkeep and repair.
• Fat-soluble and water-soluble vitamins.
• Essential minerals such as iron, calcium, and zinc.
• Foods containing plant-derived phytochemicals, which may protect against heart disease, diabetes, certain malignancies, arthritis, and osteoporosis.

A diversified diet that relies on fruits, vegetables, whole grains, legumes, dairy foods, and lean meats may provide these fundamental needs.

Kilojoules in food
In countries like Australia, kilojoules (kJ) are used to measure the amount of energy in a food or drink. (Calories (cal) are another measure of energy and is still used in certain other nations, such as the USA).
The macronutrients each offer a different amount of energy per gram:
carbohydrate = 16kJ
protein = 17kJ
fat = 37kJ
alcohol = 29kJ.

• Nutritional Food for Babies(birth to 6 months of age) (birth to 6 months of age)
Babies normally double their length and quadruple their weight between birth and one year of age. Breastmilk normally gives a newborn the needed quantities of nutrients,

water, and energy up to around 6 months of age. It is advised that newborns be solely breastfed up to roughly 6 months of age. Breast Milk is recommended over infant formula if feasible since it includes several protective and immunological elements that assist the baby's growth. Fruit juice is not suggested for infants under the age of 6 months.

Breastmilk or carefully prepared infant formula offers enough water for a healthy baby to replenish any water losses. However, all newborns require more water once solid meals are given.

• Nutritional Food for Babies(6 months and above) (6 months and above)

Solids should be started about 6 months of age to fulfill your baby's rising nutritional and developmental demands. However, nursing should continue until 12 months of age and beyond, or for as long as the mother and child choose.

Different nations have their traditions concerning which meal is more suited to start feeding a newborn. Culturally appropriate meals and preparation techniques should be supported where they are nutritionally sufficient. As a baby is progressively weaned from the breast or bottle and new meals are given, there may be decreasing body reserves of iron. To sustain nutritional body stores:

1. Give your baby meals that are high in iron and zinc, such as iron-enriched infant cereals, pureed meats, and poultry dishes, and cooked plain tofu, and legumes/soy beans/lentils. Iron-enriched rice-based cereals are commonly advised as the first meal to be given since there is the added advantage of a decreased likelihood of an allergic response.
2. Foods may be offered in any sequence, providing the texture is adequate for your baby's stage of development. Foods vary from fruits and vegetables (for vitamin and mineral content) to meat, chicken, fish, and entire eggs.

3. Do not add salt, sugar, or honey to your baby's meals. It is unneeded.
4. Avoid cow's milk as a drink in the first 12 months. Small quantities may be used in

cereals and custards. All milk used should be pasteurized.

5. Whole fruit is preferable to fruit juice. Avoid juices and sugar-sweetened drinks.

6. Put your baby to bed without a bottle, or take the bottle away when they have finished feeding to minimize long-term exposure of their teeth to sugar-containing liquids.

7. Avoid whole nuts, seeds, or similar hard foods to reduce the risk of choking.

Introduce foods one at a time. Offer new foods once every 3 to 4 days to avoid confusion and to rule out food allergy and sensitivity, feed babies during any illness, and feed up after illness. Give ample liquids if your baby has diarrhea. Cancer Council recommends that babies under 12 months are not exposed to direct sun during the daily sun protection times (when the UV Index is 3 or higher). If you are concerned about your child's vitamin D levels, see your doctor.

• Nutritional Food for young children

Once a child is eating solids, offer a wide range of foods to ensure adequate nutrition. Young children are often picky but should be encouraged to eat a wide variety of foods. Trying again with new foods may be needed for a child to accept that food. As many as 8 to 15 times may be needed.

During childhood, children tend to vary their food intake (spontaneously) to match their growth patterns. Children's food needs vary widely, depending on their growth and their level of physical activity. Like energy needs, a child's needs for protein, vitamins, and minerals increase with age. Ideally, children should be collecting stocks of nutrients in preparation for the tremendous growth surge observed throughout puberty. Acceptable weight gain and development will reveal if food consumption is appropriate.

Food-related concerns for young children include obesity, dental decay, and food sensitivity.

However, there are various suggestions to limit such occurrences, which include:

1. If a kid is acquiring incorrect weight for growth, restrict energy-dense, nutrient-poor snack foods. Increase your child's physical exercise, you might also reduce the quantity of television viewing.

2. Tooth decay may be avoided with frequent brushing and visits to the dentist. Avoid sugary meals and beverages, particularly if sticky or acidic.

3. Ensure your youngster gets adequate fluids, particularly water. Fruit juices should be minimized and soft drinks avoided.

4. Reduced-fat milk is not suggested for children under the age of 2, owing to increased energy needs and a strong growth rate at this age.

5. Be cautious of foods that may trigger allergic reactions, including peanuts, shellfish, and cow's milk. Be extremely cautious if there is a family history of food allergy.

• Nutritional Food for children approaching their teenage years

The development surge as youngsters transition into puberty demands lots of kilojoules and minerals. For females, this normally happens around 10 to 11 years of age. For males, it happens later, at roughly 12 to 13 years.

The additional energy necessary for the development and physical activity in children has to be derived from meals that also supply nutrients, instead of merely 'empty calories. Takeaway and quick meals need to be balanced with nutrient-dense foods such as wholegrain bread and cereals, fruits, legumes, nuts, vegetables, fish, and lean meats. Milk, yogurt, and cheese (mainly reduced fat) should be added to enhance calcium intake, this is particularly necessary for developing bones. Cheese should preferably be a reduced salt kind. Adolescent females should be especially encouraged to eat milk and milk products.

• Older teens and young adults

Moving out from home, beginning a job or school, and the changing lifestyle that follows the late teens and early 20s may create nutritional changes that are not necessarily favorable for overall health.

Youngsters at this stage have to be adequately advised in making an intentional effort to stay physically active, restrict alcohol consumption, and limit the number of fats and salt in their daily diet.

One needs to be cautious to include foods rich in iron and calcium and also build good eating habits that will be kept on into later life.

• Nutritional Food for pregnant women

A pregnant woman should focus on increasing her nutritional consumption, rather than her kilojoule intake, especially in the first and second trimesters. In a given nation, pregnant women are predicted to gain roughly 10 to 13 kg during pregnancy. However, this depends on the pre-pregnancy weight of the mother.

Since a nursing mother-to-be, you should not 'crash diet', as this might have a harmful influence on the baby. Eating for two should be avoided since this will lead to excessive weight gain. A healthy pregnancy only needs roughly an additional 1,400 to 1,900 kilojoules a day throughout the second and third trimester, which is similar to a glass of milk or a sandwich.

Concentrate on diet quality rather than quantity, indulge cravings but don't let them replace more healthy meals.

Nutrients for which there are increased needs during pregnancy include folate, iron, vitamin B12, and iodine. Iron is essential for oxygen transport in the body. Iron supplements might be prescribed by your doctor during pregnancy, but do not take them unless your doctor advises them. Increasing vitamin C consumption may assist enhance iron absorption from meals.

Folate is crucial 3 months before and in the first trimester of pregnancy to prevent neural tube abnormalities such as spina bifida in the infant.

All women of reproductive age should consume high-folate foods (such as green leafy vegetables, fruits, and legumes) (such as green leafy vegetables, fruits, and legumes). If preparing for pregnancy, it's vital to acquire 400 µg folate/ day and if you are pregnant, this rises to 600 µg/day. This can be gotten via a folate supplement and a diet high in folate-rich foods (remember to speak to your doctor first) (remember to talk to your doctor first). It is currently obligatory for all bread-making flour to be fortified with folic acid (a type of folate that is added to meals) (a form of folate that is added to foods).

This will help women attain their recommended consumption of folate. Iodine is necessary for the regular growth and development of the newborn. Iodine supplements are commonly prescribed during pregnancy to satisfy the increased demands since dietary sources (such as seafood, iodized salt, and bread) are unlikely to give enough iodine. Talk to your doctor about this.

The recommended consumption of calcium does not particularly increase during pregnancy. It is, however, very important that pregnant women meet calcium requirements during pregnancy.

No one knows the safe limit of alcohol intake during pregnancy. Recommendations are to not drink at all. Pregnant women are recommended to avoid foods that are connected with a greater risk of listeria bacteria (such as soft cheese and cold seafood) and to be cautious with foods that are more likely to contain mercury (such as flake) (such as flake). Listeria may badly damage your developing baby.

Being physically active has numerous advantages. If you are active and fit and are enjoying a normal pregnancy, you may continue physically active throughout your pregnancy. Otherwise, visit your doctor for guidance.
Drink lots of fluids. Do not smoke, both direct and passive smoking is connected with development retardation, higher risk of spontaneous abortion, stillbirths, placental problems, and low birth weight.

• Nutritional Food for breastfeeding mothers
Nursing women require a large amount of additional energy to deal with the demands of breastfeeding. This additional energy should come in the form of nutrient-dense meals to assist fulfill the increased dietary needs that also arise during nursing. Vegan women who are nursing (and throughout pregnancy) should take a vitamin B12 supplement.
Recommendations include:

• Eat enough food Because nursing burns off additional kilojoules.
• Eat foods that are nutrient-dense – particularly those foods that are high in folate, iodine, zinc, and calcium.
• Eat and drink frequently - breastfeeding may raise the risk of dehydration and induce constipation. Fluid demands are around 750–1000 ml a day beyond baseline needs.
• Women should continue to avoid consuming alcohol during nursing.

• Nutritional Food for menopausal women
Thinning of the bones is frequent in postmenopausal women due to hormone-related changes. At this time of a woman's life, be sure to consume foods high in calcium such as milk or, if required, take calcium supplements as suggested by a doctor. Doing more weight-bearing activities such as walking or weight training can help build bones and help maintain healthy body weight. You should also maintain a high-fiber, low-fat and low-salt diet, a diet strong in phytoestrogens has been reported to alleviate several symptoms of menopause, such as hot flushes.

Good food sources include soy products (tofu, soymilk), chickpeas, flax seeds, lentils, cracked wheat, and barley.

A range of wholegrain, nutrient-dense food, whole grains, legumes, and soy-based foods (such as tofu, soy, and linseed cereals), fruits and vegetables, and low-fat dairy products.

• Nutritional Food for elderly folks

Many individuals eat less as they become older, which might make it tougher to make sure your diet has enough diversity to incorporate all the nourishment you need. As an older person or a real adult, you need to be extra careful of your weight, so as not to get in your way of everyday living. Be as active as possible to boost your appetite and retain muscular mass.

Remain healthy with well-balanced eating and regular exercise, and eat foods that are nutrient-dense rather than energy-dense, including eggs, lean meats, fish, liver, low-fat dairy foods, nuts and seeds, legumes, fruit and vegetables, whole grain bread, and cereals.

If feasible, try to spend some time outdoors each day to improve your vitamin D synthesis for healthy bones. Limit meals that are rich in calories and poor in nutrition such as cakes, sugary biscuits, and soft drinks as well as pick foods that are naturally high in fiber to improve intestinal health. Limit the use of table salt, particularly when cooking, pick from a broad range of meals and drink appropriate water, and spend mealtimes with family and friends.

Chapter 4

WHEN YOU DON'T WATCH IT

There are numerous dangerous misunderstandings regarding weight reduction. There are no magical meals or techniques to mix foods that melt away extra body fat. To lower your weight, make incremental, doable adjustments to your lifestyle. If you're overweight, the best method to shed and maintain your weight in the long term is to modify the way you eat and improve your level of physical activity.

Understand your energy from food, when we eat, our bodies are provided with numerous nutrients. This contains vitamins, minerals, antioxidants, and energy from the macronutrients such as carbs, protein, and fat. Alcohol also gives energy; however, it is not needed for life hence it is not regarded as a real macronutrient.

Guarding Yourself Against Obesity

Fat and alcohol give far more energy per gram than both protein and carbs. A 35 g piece of bread has roughly 360kJ but 35g of butter has 1062kJ of energy, about 3 times as much as the slice of bread.

That's not to suggest fats don't constitute part of a healthful diet, because they do. What matters is the kind and quantity of fat we ingest.

Our energy demands vary based on things such as:

> age

> body size

> gender

> how active you are

> your genetics

> whether you're pregnant or nursing.

Generally speaking, the more body fat you're carrying, the larger your health risk. However, the amount of weight accumulated over your adult years also correlates to the risk. For example, a middle-aged individual who weighs 10 kg more than they did in their early 20s has an increased risk of high blood pressure, stroke, diabetes, and coronary heart disease.

Causes Of Obesity

A multitude of causes may induce obesity. Factors in childhood and adolescence are highly significant. A large percentage of obese children and adolescents grow up to be fat adults.

Factors known to raise the risk of obesity include:

• Eating more kilojoules than you use
You will acquire fat in your body if you eat more energy (kilojoules) than you utilize. Learn about balancing energy in and energy out, and good nutrition.

• Modern lifestyle
Most contemporary conveniences, such as vehicles, computers, TVs, and household appliances, diminish the need to be physically active.

• Sitting\sStudies have shown that physically active persons who spend substantial amounts of time sitting down (for example, watching TV, working at a computer, or driving) have a greater risk of obesity than those who do not sit for extended periods. Read about the hazards of sitting.

• Socioeconomic considerations
People with lower levels of education and poorer incomes are more likely to be overweight or obese.

• Changes in the food supply
Energy-dense, nutrient-poor meals, and beverages are easily accessible, aggressively advertised, and inexpensive. Portion sizes of various meals and beverages have also grown.

Hormonal Effects Of Obesity
Hormones are chemical messengers that govern activities in our bodies. They are one factor in generating obesity. The hormones leptin and insulin, sex hormones, and growth hormones regulate our hunger, metabolism (the rate at which our body consumes kilojoules for energy), and body fat distribution. People who are obese have levels of these hormones that induce improper metabolism and the storage of body fat.

A set of glands, known as the endocrine system, secretes hormones into our circulation. The endocrine system interacts with the neurological system and the immune system to assist our body deal with diverse events and pressures. Excesses or shortfalls of hormones may contribute to obesity and, on the other hand, obesity can lead to alterations in hormones.

• Obesity and leptin
The hormone leptin is created by fat cells and is released into our circulation. Leptin suppresses a person's appetite by working on certain areas of their brain to lessen their need to eat. It also appears to affect how the body controls its accumulation of body fat.
Because leptin is created by fat, leptin levels tend to be greater in persons who are obese than in those of normal weight. However, despite having larger quantities of this appetite-reducing hormone, fat persons aren't as sensitive to the effects of leptin and, as a consequence, tend not to feel full during and after a meal. The ongoing study is investigating

why leptin signals aren't getting through to the brain in fat persons.

• Obesity and insulin

Insulin, a hormone generated by the pancreas, is vital for the control of carbohydrates and the metabolism of fat. Insulin enhances glucose (sugar) absorption from the circulation in tissues such as muscles, the liver, and fat. This is a vital mechanism to ensure that energy is accessible for daily functioning and to maintain appropriate levels of circulating glucose.

In a fat person, insulin signals are occasionally lost and tissues are no longer able to manage glucose levels. This may lead to the development of type II diabetes and metabolic

The main thing is to have a balanced diet and eat enough nutrient-packed meals. It is also vital to restrict the number of calorie-packed, nutrition-poor meals to have a healthy weight.

If you consume more energy (kilojoules) than you need, you will put on weight whether those kilojoules originate from fats, carbs, or proteins. There are numerous popular myths concerning weight control, let's dispel some of them.

Chapter 5

WEIGHT MANAGEMENT

Managing your weight includes a nutritious diet and frequent exercise. Fad diets are not the solution. A healthy weight may vary for various persons. Some health issues might make it harder to regulate weight growth. Managing your weight within a healthy range may minimize your chance of acquiring health concerns.

Weight management treatments are supplied by registered practicing dietitians, GPs, commercial weight reduction programs, meal replacement programs (extremely low energy diets), and kilojoule-controlled meal programs. If you are wanting to lose weight, pick your weight management service with consideration. Some commercial weight reduction programs give healthy weight management and lifestyle guidelines to their clientele. Others may depend on untested or harmful approaches. Aiming for weight reduction may not be viable for you at this time. Ensure to visit a healthcare expert when the moment is suitable for you. Receiving expert guidance for behavioral modification may help you effectively reach your objectives.

The main thing is to have a balanced diet and eat enough nutrient-packed meals. It is also vital to restrict the number of calorie-packed, nutrition-poor meals to have a healthy weight.
If you consume more energy (kilojoules) than you need, you will put on weight whether those kilojoules originate from fats, carbs, or proteins. There are numerous popular myths concerning weight control, let's dispel some of them.

The Secret To Weight Loss
The best method to lose weight is slowly, by making tiny, manageable adjustments to your food and activity routines. Rather than becoming a slave to the number on the scales, be directed by your waist circumference - a healthy waist circumference is less than 94cm for men and less than 80cm for women.

Suggestions for safe and efficient weight reduction include:

1. Don't crash diet. You'll most likely recover the lost weight within 5 years.

2. Try to pick a range of meals that meet within the Australian Guide to Healthy Eating.

3. Be cautious of the quantities you're ingesting, the greater the serving, the more energy. This is particularly crucial for energy-dense meals and beverages such as those with high quantities of lipids and alcohol.

4. Cut down on processed and added sugars.

5. Increase your consumption of fresh fruit, veggies, and wholegrain bread and cereals.

6. Cut down or eliminate empty kilojoules from sugary beverages and alcohol.

7. Eat less takeout and snack foods.

8. Exercise for around 30 minutes on most days of the week. Introduce additional activity during your day (such as a 30-minute stroll) (such as a 30-minute walk).

9. Don't remove any food category. Instead, pick from a broad variety of meals every day and prefer 'whole', less-processed foods.

10. Have a regular plan of eating and keep to it.

11. Watch your energy (kilojoule) intake.

12. Ultimately, to minimize weight gain, energy intake should not be higher than energy output.

13. Avoiding big portion sizes and restricting consumption of saturated fats and added sweets can assist to keep your energy intake in balance.

14. Regular exercise is also crucial for long-term weight reduction success.

If you are not sure where to start or find it difficult to maintain your weight, get guidance from a dietician. Dietitians can lead you to a healthy way of eating that is based on the latest research and adapted to fit your health and lifestyle.

Talk to your GP about weight management services

Your GP understands your medical history and may either discuss proper weight reduction measures or refer to an approved practicing dietician.

It's crucial to talk with your GP before beginning any weight reduction program. This is particularly crucial if you use any sort of prescription medication or if you have a pre-existing ailment, such as:

>Obesity

>All kinds of diabetes include type 1, type 2, and gestational

>Pregnancy or breastfeeding

>Kidney problems

>Liver conditions

>Food allergies

>Digestive system diseases such as celiac disease

>High blood pressure (hypertension)

>Heart conditions, angina or cardiac arrhythmia

And so many more health concerns you might be suffering.

Also, registered practicing dietitians are acknowledged specialists who can give expert nutrition and dietary guidance. Dietitians can lead you to excellent food and health knowledge that is relevant to your requirements.

Generally speaking, a decent weight management service will:

i. Aim to enhance general health, such as decreasing blood cholesterol, and reducing your risk of type 2 diabetes and heart disease.

ii. Encourage a balanced approach to eat, incorporating foods from all of the basic food categories and in appropriate portion amounts.

iii. Cater to your unique wants.

iv. Focus on lowering body fat (for example, waist measurement), not merely total body weight.

v. Include frequent exercise and physical activity, most days of the week.

vi. Advise on how to enhance long-term eating and exercise habits.

vii. Offer continued help with your weight control, even after you have attained your goal weight.

viii. Give explicit information about the return policy.

Don't employ a weight management service that encourages you to:\s• Cut out one or more of the main dietary categories.

• Replace meals with powders or supplements.

• Encourage short-term adjustments to eat behavior rather than longer-term, sustainable improvements.

• Use untested or hazardous equipment such as saunas, passive exercise machines, diuretics, and body wraps.
• Focus on quick weight reduction, but doesn't contain any information on how to maintain a healthy weight in the long run.

Consult with social media sites for weight control and health guidance.
If you decide to start a very low energy diet (VLED) utilizing meal replacement shakes, bars or soups, visit a nutritionist to make sure you:

>Are you still fulfilling all your nutritional requirements?
>Have continuing assistance to complete the program.
>Have access to counsel for returning to your usual eating pattern to reduce severe weight regain.
>Choosing a kilojoule-controlled food service.

Our dietary demands fluctuate with various life stages. To stay fit and healthy, it is vital to take into consideration the increased demands put on your body by these changes.

To satisfy your body's normal nutritional demands, you should consume:

• A broad array of healthful foods
• Water on a regular basis
• Enough kilojoules for energy, with carbs as the preferable source
• Essential fatty acids from meals such as oily fish, almonds, avocado
• Adequate protein for cell maintenance and repair
• Fat-soluble and water-soluble vitamins
• Essential minerals such as iron, calcium, and zinc
• Foods containing plant-derived phytochemicals, which may protect against heart disease, diabetes, certain cancers, arthritis, and osteoporosis.

A diversified diet that relies on fruits, vegetables, whole grains, legumes, dairy foods, and lean meats may provide these fundamental needs.